Gisela Maria de Figueiredo

Exposure to Pesticides and Long-Term Health Effects

Gisela Maria de Figueiredo

Exposure to Pesticides and Long-Term Health Effects

Cross-sectional study of 370 rural workers exposed to pesticides over the long term

ScienciaScripts

To God for enlightening and supporting me in life's difficult moments.

To my parents, Antonio and Cleonice, for their unconditional love and support.

To my siblings, Cíntia and Eduardo, for their friendship and encouragement.

To Jaime for his love, companionship and patience.

Without you this work would not be possible...

ACKNOWLEDGEMENTS

To Prof Dr Ângelo Zanaga Trapé, for his guidance, trust, friendship and the opportunity to carry out this work.

To the members of the qualification committee, Prof. Dr. Sérgio Roberto de Lucca, for his availability, advice and pertinent suggestions, to Prof. Dr. Carlos Roberto Silveira Corrêa, for his valuable criticism and contributions to the finalisation of this work.

My work colleagues, Carina and Siomara, for their friendship, encouragement and support during this difficult stage.

To the statistician Hélio Rubens de Carvalho Nunes, for his great help in the statistical analyses of this work and for his always constructive criticism.

To the secretary of the Postgraduate Programme in Collective Health, Maisa, for her attention and for always being available to help.

To the staff of the SAM-HC Unicamp, for their help in sorting the patient records.

To my sister, confidante and teacher, Cíntia, for her great contributions and example to follow.

My mum, Cleonice, and the proofreader, Elaine F. A. Corradello, for their help with the spelling and grammar of this work.

To Teresinha Baratella, for her help with the translations.

To all the patients and rural workers seen at Unicamp's Toxicology Outpatient Clinic who trusted us and allowed us to carry out this study.

"Knowledge is proud to have learnt so much;

wisdom is humble because it doesn't know any better"

(William Cowper)

SUMMARY

The use of pesticides has had a serious impact on the environment and especially on public health, with reports of contamination of various media (air, water and soil) and cases of acute poisoning and death, but few real reports of the chronic effects of long-term exposure to these substances. The aim of this study was to assess the health effects of workers who had been exposed to pesticides in the long term and who were treated at the Toxicology Outpatient Clinic at Unicamp's Hospital de Clínicas in 2006 and 2007. This is a descriptive cross-sectional observational study that reports and analyses the effects on the health of 370 workers occupationally exposed to pesticides over the long term. The variables studied in these patients were: age, gender, work relationship, type of contact with pesticides, use of personal protective equipment, how they were referred to the outpatient clinic, length of exposure to pesticides, type of exposure to pesticides, alterations found on physical and laboratory examination and diagnosis. These variables were collected from the patients' medical records. Excel was used to set up the database and create the variables, and SPSS version 15 was used to statistically analyse the data. In this way, we tried to establish whether workers exposed to pesticides over the long term, within the studied regional reality of pesticide use, developed chronic damage to their health.

Keywords: long-term exposure to pesticides, rural workers, health effects.

SUMMARY

CHAPTER 1

INTRODUCTION

1.1- Definition of pesticides

There are several names given to these chemical substances in the literature. In English, this group of chemical products is called "pesticides" or "agrochemicals" and can be defined as any substance used to kill or, conversely, control pests (The National Environmental Education & Training Foundation, 2003). It should be noted that the Portuguese word pesticida, translated as pesticide, is often used as a synonym for agrotoxic. However, this translation is erroneous, since peste in Portuguese does not mean plague (Alonzo and Corrêa, 2003). In Spanish, such products are called "plaguicidas", i.e. pesticides. In Brazil, the name "pesticides" was used until the creation of federal law 7802 in June 1989, which called them agrotoxics (Tomazin, 2007).

In this study, we chose to use the term pesticides, as this is the term currently used in Brazilian legislation.

Pesticides and related products are defined by Decree No. 4074 of January 2002, which regulates Law No. 7802, as:

> "Products and components of physical, chemical or biological processes intended for use in the production, storage and processing of agricultural products, in pastures, in the protection of native or established forests and other ecosystems and urban, water and industrial environments, whose purpose is to alter the composition of flora and fauna in order to preserve it from the harmful action of living beings considered harmful, as well as substances and products used as defoliants, desiccants, growth stimulators and inhibitors."

According to the Council on Scientific Affairs (1997), agrochemicals cover a diverse group of chemical and biological agents that are intentionally used in the environment to selectively control plants, animals and microorganisms.

organisms. In public health, they are usually used in vector control programmes, such as insects and rodents. In agriculture, they are used to control insects, weeds and micro-organisms that can damage the growth or harvest of crops.

1.1- A historical approach to the use of agrochemicals in the world:

The use of chemical substances to eliminate pests dates back to antiquity. The Greeks and Romans used sulphur to combat pests. Other substances such as calcium hydroxide, pyrethrum (extracted from chrysanthemum flowers and historically used by Caucasian tribes), as well as arsenic and lime, were used during the 19th century to combat insects and fungi (Alonzo, 1995; Gallo, 1996; Peres, 1999; Plimmer, 2001; Nishiyama, 2003; Alonzo and Corrêa, 2003; Silva et al, 1999).

In the mid-1920s, Mueller discovered the insecticide DDT - dichlorodiphenyltrichlorethane, and several other organochlorines, as well as hexachlorobenzene and hexachlorocyclohexane, resulting in the extensive use of insecticides at the end of that decade. The insecticide DDT was developed to control insect-borne diseases, and the herbicide Phenoxy to increase food production (Gallo, 1996; Plimmer, 2001).

In the mid-1930s, Willy Lange and Gerhard Schrader discovered a new chemical group, the organophosphates, and devoted much effort to elucidating their mechanism of action (Gallo, 1996; Plimmer, 2001).

The use of pesticides intensified even after World War II, in the 1950s (Gallo, 1996; Peres, 1999; Araújo et al. 2000; Kotaka, 2000). Their use was justified by the discourse of population growth, hunger and the need to produce food on a large scale, and even to meet market needs (Oliveira, 2004). Until the mid-1950s, inorganic substances were used to control pests and, after the Second World War, synthetic substances were introduced onto the market for this purpose, giving rise to various new compounds.

In the subsequent decades (60s, 70s and 80s), the pesticides developed became increasingly specific based on the chemical, physical and biological mechanisms of living beings (Alonzo, 1995; Gallo, 1996; Peres, 1999; Kotaka, 2000; Plimmer, 2001).

In this way, the 20th century was characterised, among other things, by an intense and continuous process of technological and organisational change, which hit the world of production hard and led to major transformations in the forms, processes and working relationships. Agriculture, which for centuries had been the livelihood of farmers and their families, became an activity geared towards commercial production. Behind this change was the need to feed an ever-growing population, which according to the United Nations will number 7.9 billion people by 2025 (ILO, 2001).

1.2- A historical approach to pesticide use in Brazil

In Brazil, the use of pesticides began in the 1940s (Alonzo, 1995; Silva, 2004), with the first pesticide introduced being HCH (hexachlorocyclohexane) in 1946, followed by DDT, parathion and toxaphene (Araújo et al., 2000; Nishiyama, 2003).

But it was from the 1960s onwards that pesticides definitely became part of rural workers' daily lives, thus increasing the risks to which they were already exposed. However, it was from 1975 onwards, with the National Development Plan (PND), which aimed to open up Brazil to international trade in these products, that there was a real boom in the use of pesticides in rural labour. Under the terms of the PND, farmers were obliged to buy these products in order to obtain rural credit. Each loan applied for had to include a set quota of agrochemicals (Garcia, 1996; Meirelles, 1996; Sayad, 1984) and this obligation, together with the manufacturers' advertising, led to a huge increase and spread in the use of agrochemicals in Brazil (Garcia, 1996).

The indiscriminate use of pesticides in Brazil was due to the replacement of subsistence agriculture by export agriculture, the need to protect crops from resistant pests and the need to combat vectors of endemic diseases (Nishiyama, 2003).

A certain evolution of agriculture can be considered to have occurred through its modernisation, since farmers no longer depend exclusively on the natural fertility of the soil and rudimentary and predatory production techniques to grow crops. However, the intense use of natural resources and pesticides has aggravated pre-existing environmental problems, leading to changes in agricultural policies and favouring the current phase of Brazilian agriculture: sustainable agriculture (Nishiyama, 2003).

In Latin America, Brazil is currently the largest consumer of pesticides (Moreira et al., 2002; Silva, 2004).

Considering the national market, Peres et al. (2001) stated that developing countries are responsible for 20% of the world pesticide market, with Brazil accounting for the equivalent of 1.1 billion dollars or 150,000 tonnes/year.

According to the National Union of the Agricultural Defence Products Industry (SINDAG), in 2001 Brazil was the eighth largest consumer of these products in the world, with 3.2 Kg/ha of pesticides. Also according to SINDAG, in 2003 there were 648 products on the market in Brazil, 34.4% of which were insecticides, 30.8% herbicides, 22.8% fungicides, 4.9% acaricides and 7.1% other chemical groups.

Brazil is currently the second largest pesticide market in the world, with sales of around US$ 5.4 billion in 2007, just behind the United States with US$ 7.7 billion. Sales of pesticides rose by 36% between January and August 2008, compared to the same period last year (ANDEF, 2008).

1.3- Classification of pesticides

Pesticides can be classified in different ways. In this study, the classifications are discussed: according to the pest to be controlled, the chemical group and the type of formulation or presentation.

Depending on the pest you want to control, these can be: insecticides, acaricides or ticks, fungicides, soil fumigants and nematicides, herbicides, growth regulators, rodenticides and molluscicides (Almeida, 1995; Fernandes, 1970).

Classification according to chemical group consists of: bipyridyls, carbamates, organochlorine compounds, organophosphorus compounds, thiazine derivatives, phenoxyacetic acid derivatives, chloronitrophenol derivatives, pyrethroids, dithiocarbamates, others such as organotins and mercurials (Almeida, 1995; Fernandes, 1970).

Classification according to the type of formulation or presentation refers to the way in which the ingredients are combined for sale and use. It includes the percentage of each active ingredient (the chemical intended to kill a pest), coadjuvant agents (which provide additional properties to the product), solvents, adhesives and humectants (to give greater hold to insects and leaves); other characteristics such as its physical state: liquid, powder or granules, and the way it will be mixed before application (Bull and Hathaway, 1986; Fernandes, 1970).

1.4- Toxic effects of pesticides

Pesticides include a wide variety of chemical products with significant differences in absorption, distribution, biotransformation, elimination and site of action. These characteristics directly influence toxicity to humans (Alonzo, 1995).

The main groups of pesticides and those most frequently associated with acute and chronic poisoning are described below:

1.4.1- Organophosphate insecticides

Insecticides cause the most poisoning and a large number of deaths in the country.

These insecticides are well absorbed through the skin and by ingestion, and very little by inhalation. It is important to note that more than 90% of absorption occurs through the skin and the rest through digestion, as the droplets from sprays are not inhalable because they are large and end up being swallowed when they are in the upper airways (Trapé, 2003).

The mechanism of action of organophosphate insecticides is associated with the inhibition of acetylcholinesterase (AChE) in nerve tissues, allowing the accumulation of free ACh. Signs of toxicity result from stimulation of muscarinic receptors in the parasympathetic autonomic nervous system, stimulation and blockade of nicotinic receptors (including sympathetic and parasympathetic ganglia), as well as the neuromuscular junction plate, in addition to those resulting from effects on the central nervous system (Echobicon, 1993; Fernandes, 1970).

Three characteristic syndromes have been identified: the first is often associated with exposure to high concentrations of insecticides, with effects that can persist for months after exposure, involving neuroconductive, cognitive and neuromuscular functions. The second, also called "intermediate syndrome", is characterised by neurological signs and symptoms that appear within 24-96 hours of the acute cholinergic crisis. The latter presents a delayed neuropathy that appears 2-5 weeks after the acute phase of intoxication, resulting from the phosphorylation and inhibition of the so-called neurotoxic esterase, NTE (Echobicon, 1993).

Other serious and little-mentioned effects of long-term exposure are related to blood clotting disorders that some organophosphates can cause, often leading to the death of the contaminated person (Trapé, 2003).

A current toxicological suspicion refers to the possibility of long-term exposure causing psychological alterations and depression with a risk of suicide attempts. This hypothesis has been investigated, but so far the studies are inconclusive (Rosenstokl et al. 1991; Faria et al.,1990)

1.4.2- Carbamate insecticides

Carbamic insecticides are direct inhibitors of acetylcholinesterase. This enzyme becomes carbamylated, leading to the accumulation of free ACh, and finally the organism manifests signs and symptoms similar to those caused by organophosphates. The inhibition is characterised as labile, reversible and short-lived, because the carbamylesterase hydrolyses quickly and completely, resulting in the reactivation of the inhibited enzyme (Fernandes, 1970).

1.4.3- Pyrethroid insecticides

This group has been widely used not only in farming, but also to combat the dengue vector and in domestic environments (Trapé, 2003).

They are synthetic compounds similar to pyrethrins, used in agriculture and in the home.

They are non-systemic contact insecticides, of which there are more than 2,000 trade names. They are substances that stimulate the central nervous system by prolonging the opening time of sodium channels in the nerve membrane, and are less toxic to mammals than to insects. However, hypersensitivity reactions and prolongation of the period of nervous excitability have been described in farmers (Ellenhorn and Barceloux, 1988).

In acute poisoning, they can cause irritation of the mucous membranes, nausea, vomiting and diarrhoea. Because they are sensitising, they can cause skin and upper airway allergies, such as acute bronchitis due to sensitisation.

In long-term exposure, these products can cause peripheral neuritis and haematological alterations such as leucopenia (Trapé, 2003).

1.4.4- Organochlorine insecticides

The use of most organochlorines is banned in the country due to their high persistence in the environment and their ability to accumulate in living beings, especially humans, as well as their carcinogenic effect on laboratory animals (Trapé, 2003).

They are pesticides used in agriculture and public health to control vectors. These compounds have prolonged persistence in the environment, as well as relative neutrality and high solubility in adipose tissue (Garcia and Almeida, 1991). They stimulate the central nervous system by having a direct effect on the neuronal membrane, especially the axon. DDT, in particular, affects sodium channels, prolonging their opening time and therefore increasing the flow of the ion through the membrane. Other organochlorines, such as Lindane, inhibit gamma-amino butyric acid (GABA), causing stimulation of the central nervous system through the release of neurotransmitters. Endusulfan acts on the activity of the Calmomodulin-Ca++ dependent ATPase, also by altering the serotoninergic system and inhibiting GABA receptors (Fernandes, 1970; Tordoir and Sittert, 1994).

These pesticides act directly on the organs, especially the central nervous system, producing muscle contractions, tingling (tongue, lips, face and hands), tremors, convulsions and coma. Seizures are extremely serious.

In long-term exposure, cardiac alterations can occur, such as heart rhythm disorders, liver and kidney alterations, as well as behavioural disorders (Trapé, 2003).

1.4.5- Fungicides

Among fungicides, several groups have already presented toxicological problems, such as mercurials, hexachlorobenzene and captafol. However, they are banned and therefore no longer used in the country.

The most toxicologically relevant fungicides today are dithiocarbamates. These products are widely used on tomato, strawberry, fig and flower crops, among others, and, from the point of view of acute poisoning, present symptoms and signs of mucous membrane irritation, such as conjunctivitis, rhinitis and pharyngitis. Nausea, vomiting and diarrhoea can accompany the acute condition.

In long-term exposure, because some of these fungicides contain manganese in their molecule, they can cause a type of Parkinsonism, with tremors of the extremities that can evolve into an irreversible condition (Trapé, 2003).

1.5.6- Glyphosate herbicide

In reality, this product does not present major toxicological problems, despite being an organophosphate, but it is not an enzyme inhibitor like insecticides. There is a commercial formulation that has a surfactant substance that has an important dermatological irritant action, which is not an action of the active ingredient itself. As this is the most commercialised formulation in the country, it is necessary to be aware of this risk (Trapé, 2003).

1.5.7- Paraquat herbicide

A contact and desiccant herbicide of the bipyridyl class, widely used in agriculture and also of great importance in public health. The mechanism of toxic action involves the reduction of simple electrons in the herbicide to free radical species. The herbicide's free radicals are oxidised by cellular oxygen, producing superoxide anion and other oxygen radicals in a continuous redox reaction. Paraquat is known to be responsible for a large number of acute poisonings and deaths resulting from multisystem failure (pulmonary, renal, hepatic, cardiac and adrenal) or progressive pulmonary fibrosis 5 to 14 days after exposure (Ellenhorn and Barceloux, 1988).

It is a herbicide that is well absorbed via the digestive tract, can be absorbed through irritated or damaged skin and the inhalation route is the least absorbent (Trapé, 2003).

1.5.8- Herbicide 2,4 D

This product is widely used throughout the country on sugar cane and pastures. It is well absorbed through the skin, digestive tract and inhalation, acutely causing transient changes in glycaemia, which can simulate a

clinical picture of diabetes, as well as neuromuscular alterations due to peripheral neuritis, which is an inflammatory process of the long nerves of the lower and upper limbs.

For long-term effects, the concern is with dioxins, which are technical impurities that may be present in these products. Dioxins are persistent organochlorine substances that are suspected of causing damage to germ cells, which could lead to reproductive disorders and some types of cancer such as lymphomas, which are on the rise in terms of the world population (Trapé, 2003).

1.5.9- Rat poison

Currently, rodenticides are based on anticoagulants, the dicoumarins, which are well absorbed by the digestive tract and can cause various degrees of haemorrhage in acute poisoning, depending on the dose ingested. The group most at risk in this case are children who come into contact with these substances in the form of bait, some of which simulate treats that are very attractive to children (Trapé, 2003).

Multiple or combined exposure

The rural working population is hardly ever exposed to a single type of pesticide, but there is a multiplicity of exposures to the various groups already mentioned in a systematic and long-term manner, with acute episodes of intoxication by one of the specific groups. Therefore, the great challenge for Toxicology in the coming decades will be to assess individuals with multiple exposures over many years (Trapé, 2003).

For some time now, researchers in other countries have noted various adverse effects of this type of exposure (Kaloyanova, 1983). Table 1 shows this diversity of effects on the systems of the human organism. It is important to note that there is no definition of a specific group of agrochemicals, but rather a synergistic action between them, which constitutes a situation of considerable concern in terms of public health.

Table 1- Effects of chronic exposure to multiple pesticides

ORGAN/SYSTEM	EFFECT
Nervous system	Astheno-vegetative syndrome, vegetative polyneuritis radiculitis, encephalopathies, dysencephalitis, vegetative vascular dystonia, cerebral sclerosis, retrobulbar neuritis with visual acuity, retinal angiopathy.
Respiratory system	Chronic tachyitis, initial pneumofibrosis, pulmonary emphysema,

	bronchial asthma.
Cardiovascular system	Chronic toxic myocarditis, chronic coronary insufficiency, hypertension, hypotension.
Liver	Chronic hepatitis, cholecystitis, impaired detoxification and other functions.
Kidneys	Albuminuria, nicturia, disturbances in urea, nitrogen and creatinine clearance.
Gastrointestinal tract	Chronic gastritis, duodenitis, ulcers, chronic colitis (haemorrhagic, spastic and polypoid formations), hypersecretion and hyperacidity, impaired motor skills.
Haematopoietic system	Leucopenia, changes in reticulocytes and lymphocytes, eosinopenia, monocytosis, changes in haemoglobin
Skin	Dermatitis and eczema
Eyes	Conjunctivitis and blepharitis.

Finally, it is important to emphasise that most of the time the symptoms of people exposed to pesticides are vague and non-objective, such as headaches, dizziness, malaise, weakness and stomach pain. It is therefore necessary to pay attention to this situation so that there is a suspicion of effects caused by pesticides and not by diseases of other origins that can also present non-specific symptoms and affect people exposed to these poisons (Trapé, 2003).

1.6- The Toxicology Outpatient Clinic at Unicamp's Hospital de Clínicas

The Toxicology Outpatient Clinic at Unicamp's Hospital de Clínicas serves the entire Campinas region, with an estimated population of 2,633,523 million people (IBGE, 2007). It is of fundamental importance within the care structure of the Unified Health System (SUS), also treating patients referred from other regions of the state of São Paulo and from various other states in the country, functioning, in fact, as a tertiary reference centre, at state and national levels (Trapé, 1995).

The Toxicology Outpatient Clinic has been operating since 1984, after the Poison Control Centre (CCI) was set up. It deals with regional referrals of cases that do not require hospitalisation, and carries out outpatient monitoring after the discharge of patients hospitalised for poisoning problems in general. Referrals can come from the regional health services, from the JRC on duty, or from the HC Emergency Room through active search, fieldwork carried out by professionals from the Toxicology Outpatient Clinic, together with 5th year interns from the Unicamp School of Medicine, as a practical activity in the Environmental Health subject and as part of a teaching and care programme.

The active search is carried out every fortnight in various locations in the Campinas region. In this fieldwork, various populations are interviewed by 5th year students from Unicamp's

Faculty of Medicine, using an investigation form (Appendix I) and cholinesterase testing using the Edson method.

In the pesticide exposure investigation form, patients are first asked about their general data, working conditions and use of pesticides. They are then assessed on epidemiological data, clinical condition and the result of the Edson cholinesterase test is noted.

The criteria used to refer interviewees to the clinic are threefold: the epidemiological criterion, if the farmer has already been hospitalised for pesticide poisoning less than 10 years ago; the clinical criterion if he reports symptoms of possible poisoning and the laboratory criterion if he has an acetylcholinesterase activity of 75% or less in the Edson test.

Farmers who don't meet the criteria for being referred to the clinic are given advice on the risks of using pesticides and the need to use personal protective equipment (PPE). Those who are referred will undergo a more detailed clinical investigation at the Toxicology Outpatient Clinic, where a full physical examination will be carried out and laboratory tests from the clinic's protocol will be requested.

The laboratory tests in the Toxicology Outpatient Clinic protocol are markers of exposure and health effects in patients exposed to pesticides.

This is why the Elman cholinesterase test is requested, which is more specific than the Edson test requested during the active search. This method quantifies plasma and erythrocyte cholinesterase, thus demonstrating whether there is any decrease in acetylcholinesterase activity and whether this is due to the plasma or erythrocyte component. The other tests requested are: blood count, kidney profile (A1M and MICROALB) and liver profile (AST, ALT, GGT and FALC), which will show whether the patient has lesions in the main organs targeted by the pesticides, which are bone marrow, kidneys and liver respectively. Electroneuromyography is also requested if the patient presents peripheral neurological alterations on physical examination. Other tests may be ordered later, depending on the results found in these initial protocol tests.

At the Toxicology Outpatient Clinic, patients will be seen and monitored by 4th and 5th year medical students, who are supervised by an Environmental Health doctor, an occupational health doctor, a health nurse and a biologist. The clinic is open in the afternoons on Tuesdays and Thursdays on the 3rd floor of Unicamp's Hospital de Clínicas.

Thus, the HC Unicamp Toxicology Outpatient Clinic acts as a regional reference service for the assessment of individuals exposed to or contaminated by pesticides, seeking to investigate and establish a relationship between the diseases detected and exposure to pesticides.

A more formal service was therefore organised to care for the population exposed to these products, from an outpatient point of view, as a specialised secondary level reference, with local and regional coverage, as part of the proposed action of a Health Surveillance Programme for Populations Exposed to Pesticides in the Campinas region (Trappé, 1995).

CHAPTER 2

JUSTIFICATIONS

Pesticides are one of the most important risk factors for human health. Used on a large scale by various productive sectors and more intensely by the agricultural sector, they have been the subject of various types of studies, both because of the damage they cause to the health of human populations, and workers in particular, and because of the damage to the environment and the emergence of resistance in target organisms (pests and vectors). In agriculture, they are widely used in large-scale monoculture systems. The crops that use them most are soya, sugar cane, maize, coffee, citrus fruit, irrigated rice and cotton. Less significant crops in terms of planted area, such as tobacco, grapes, strawberries, potatoes, tomatoes and other vegetables and fruit, also use large quantities of pesticides (ILO, 2001; Brazil, 1997).

The main exposure to these products occurs in the agricultural sector, public health, disinsection companies, transport, marketing and production of pesticides. In addition to occupational exposure, food and environmental contamination puts other population groups at risk of poisoning. These include farmers' families, the population surrounding a production unit and the general population, who eat what is produced in the countryside.

It can be said that the effects of pesticides on health do not only concern exposed workers, but the population in general. As Berlinguer aptly puts it, the production unit doesn't just affect the worker, but infects the environment and has repercussions on society as a whole (Chediack, 1986).

Farmers' difficulty in accessing health centres, professionals' lack of preparation to relate health problems to work in general and exposure to pesticides in particular, incorrect diagnoses, the scarcity of biological monitoring laboratories and the lack of early and/or reliable biomarkers are some of the factors that influence underdiagnosis and underreporting. Therefore, it can be said that the official Brazilian data on pesticide poisoning does not reflect the seriousness of the Brazilian reality, as can be seen in the studies by Freitas et al. (1986), Peres et al. (2001), Moreira et al. (2002), among others.

The few actions aimed at valuing social and environmental relations, especially with regard to work environments, and the lack of epidemiological knowledge of occupational poisoning, make it difficult to define strategies that can effectively establish strict control of these diseases.

Despite the efforts of various international organisations and the investment of industries and governments, the vast majority of chemical products have still not been fully and adequately studied. The massive production of chemical substances, combined with their intense and often indiscriminate use, has taken its toll on society and the environment, with important repercussions on public and environmental health (Zambrone, 1992).

With few exceptions, the late effects of pesticides on human health are difficult to detect. The health risks may be so small that they are below the detection power of epidemiological studies, and it is also possible that false positive associations may be observed. However, there is no doubt about the need to investigate the morbid effects on humans of exposure to pesticides (Silva, 2004).

Generally, acute poisonings with immediate effects are recognised without difficulty due to the short period between contact with the toxic substance and the appearance of signs and symptoms. Late effects are more difficult to associate with exposure, due to the time that has passed or the appearance of more subtle or atypical disorders, or both (Morris, 1998).

Information indicating the possibility of chronic health effects following exposure is based mainly on laboratory animals, with little epidemiological evidence in humans (Garcia, 2001).

The first information on health problems related to pesticides in Brazil dates back to 1950, when the Biological Institute of the State Department of Agriculture found cases of illness in 118 cotton farmers in the Presidente Prudente region, with 21 deaths from a product called Paratiom, an organophosphate insecticide (PLanet, 1950; Rodrigues et al.,1957; Almeida,1967).

In the 1970s and 1980s, states such as Paraná and Rio Grande do Sul began to identify environmental and health problems caused by pesticides, indicating the increasing use of these products in the country's main agricultural production regions (Siqueira, 1983; Paraná State Health Department, 1983).

With the establishment of Poison Control Centres in various Brazilian states from the 1980s onwards, the reporting of pesticide-related illnesses became more systematised and a National Toxic-Pharmacological Information System (SINITOX) was set up, which consolidates the data generated in the various states of the country and is coordinated by the Ministry of Health's Oswaldo Cruz Foundation, which publishes annual statistics on poisoning cases recorded by Poison Control Centres.

In 2006, a total of 107,958 poisonings were recorded in SINITOX, and 6,588 (6.10%) were classified as occupational. Of the occupational poisonings, 1,874 (28.4%) were recorded as being caused by pesticides and the like, coming in second place as an occupational cause, behind only poisonings caused by venomous animals (SINITOX, 2006).

By analysing current SINITOX data, it can be concluded that the problems caused by pesticides are not only a health problem for farmers, but also a serious public health problem (Alonzo, 2000). This conclusion is reached by analysing only the cases reported by Poison Control Centres, which are only those considered to be acute intoxications, which occur suddenly and often have a dramatic outcome. This analysis does not include cases of long-term adverse effects, which are now the most worrying for professionals working in the field of environmental health and toxicology.

CHAPTER 3

OBJECTIVES

3.1- General objective

     - To study the effects on the health of workers who were exposed to pesticides in the long term and who were treated at the Toxicology Outpatient Clinic of the Unicamp Hospital de Clínicas in 2006 and 2007.

3.2- Specific objectives

- To trace the profile of rural workers exposed to pesticides in the long term, treated at the HC Unicamp toxicology clinic in 2006 and 2007.

- Describe the alterations in the physical and laboratory examinations found in the patients studied.

- To analyse the association between gender, age, alcohol consumption, the presence of metabolic alterations, the type of referral, the work relationship, combined exposure to pesticides, the type of contact with pesticides and the use of personal protective equipment (PPE) and the alterations found in the health of these workers.

- To study the effect of exposure time to pesticides on the occurrence of alterations found in the health of exposed workers.

CHAPTER 4

SUBJECTS AND METHODS

4.1- Subjects

Patients with long-term occupational exposure to pesticides seen at the Toxicology Outpatient Clinic of the Unicamp Hospital de Clínicas in 2006 and 2007.

4.2- Methods

4.2.1- Type of study

This is a descriptive cross-sectional observational study that reports and analyses the effects on the health of 370 workers occupationally exposed to pesticides over the long term who were treated at the HC Unicamp toxicology clinic in 2006 and 2007.

4.2.2- Study scenario

The Toxicology Outpatient Clinic at Unicamp's Hospital de Clínicas was chosen as the setting for this study. It has been treating patients referred from various medical services since 1984 and is a regional and national reference in the care of workers occupationally exposed to pesticides.

4.2.3- Population

All 370 patients seen at the Toxicology Outpatient Clinic at Unicamp's Hospital de Clínicas in 2006 and 2007 were studied.

4.2.4- Data collection

Data was collected by analysing the medical records of 370 patients seen at the Toxicology Outpatient Clinic of the Hospital das Clínicas at Unicamp in 2006 and 2007.

The variables studied in these patients were age, gender, the presence of behavioural and organic factors such as alcoholism and metabolic alterations, the work relationship, the type of contact with pesticides, the use of personal protective equipment, the way they were referred to the clinic, the length of exposure to pesticides, the presence of combined exposure to pesticides, the alterations found on physical examination and in the laboratory, and the diagnosis.

With regard to the variables alcoholism and metabolic alterations, the patient was considered an alcoholic if they reported drinking more than 20g of alcohol per week and with metabolic alterations if they had any metabolic disease (dyslipidaemia, obesity, thyroid dysfunction, diabetes and/or plurimetabolic syndrome) during the anamnesis.

With regard to the working relationship variable, the patients studied were classified as owners, sharecroppers, free-lancers, salaried workers and others (when they had a working relationship that did not include the others).

With regard to the type of contact, the workers were categorised into two groups. Direct contact was when the farmer applied, prepared or diluted the pesticide and when he washed the clothes used in the application. Indirect contact was related to planting, harvesting, disbudding, packaging, pruning and weeding.

The Personal Protective Equipment surveyed included wearing long trousers, a long-sleeved shirt, suitable waterproof clothing, closed shoes or boots, suitable boots, gloves, goggles, masks, hats or caps.

As for how workers were referred to the HC-Unicamp Toxicology Outpatient Clinic, it was through active search (fieldwork carried out by the Environmental Health discipline), referrals from other HC-Unicamp specialities, referrals from the JRC-Unicamp and referrals from other Regional Health Centres.

The time of exposure to pesticides variable took into account the total time of exposure to these chemical substances throughout the working life of the worker studied.

With regard to the variable presence of combined exposure, this was considered positive when the farmer used more than one chemical group of pesticide and negative when he didn't or didn't know the type of pesticide he used.

The alterations found in the physical examination of the patients studied were taken from their medical records. All the patients underwent a complete and thorough physical examination by the 4º and 5º year medical students who attended them during their visits to the Toxicology Outpatient Clinic, under the supervision of the teaching staff. In this way, the alterations observed were described.

The laboratory tests assessed were those requested by the Toxicology Outpatient Clinic protocol, which are markers of exposure and health effects resulting from contact with pesticides. These tests include the haemogram to assess bone marrow function; the liver profile which consists of assessing AST (aspartate transaminase aminotransferase), ALT (alanine transaminase aminotransferase), GGT (gamma glutamyltransferase) and FA (alkaline phosphatase); The renal profile, which assesses A1M (alpha 1 microglobulin), a marker of early tubular renal damage, and MICROALB (microalbuminuria), a marker of early glomerular renal damage, and the cholinesterase test, which consists of an acetylcholinesterase test using the Elman method, specifying the value of plasma and erythrocyte cholinesterases.

An ENMG (electroneuromyography) was also requested as a complementary test when the patient showed alterations during his peripheral neurological physical examination.

With regard to diagnosis, two groups of patients were established. Those who had no alterations in the physical examination and/or laboratory tests were classified as "Long-term exposure to pesticides", since all the patients studied had been exposed to pesticides for at least one year. Patients who showed alterations in their physical examination and/or laboratory tests that made them think of some chronic damage to their health were classified as "Health effects". The term "chronic pesticide intoxication" was not used since the criteria for defining this diagnosis are still much debated in the literature.

4.2.5- Data processing and analysis

Microsoft Excel® was used to set up the database and create the variables, and SPSS® version 15 was used to carry out the statistical analysis of this data.

4.2.6- Statistical methodology

Firstly, the profile of the rural workers seen at the HC Unicamp Toxicology Outpatient Clinic in 2006 and 2007 was analysed in terms of age, gender, alcohol consumption, presence of metabolic alterations, how they were referred to the clinic, work relationship, type of contact with pesticides and the presence of combined exposure.

In the second stage, a descriptive analysis was made of the alterations in the physical and laboratory examinations found in the patients studied and the diagnoses made.

Subsequently, the effect of each variable studied on changes in the physical examination, laboratory tests and diagnoses was analysed, checking for any variables that could interfere with the results of this study.

Finally, the effect of exposure time to pesticides on the occurrence of alterations in physical and laboratory examinations and on diagnoses was studied.

4.2.7- Ethical aspects

No volunteers took part in this research. The research data was collected by reviewing the medical records of patients seen at the Toxicology Outpatient Clinic in 2006 and 2007. There was therefore no reason to use an Informed Consent Form (ICF).

No vulnerable groups were involved in this study either, as all the patients seen at the outpatient clinic were workers, of legal age and had decision-making capacity.

In this type of research, there were no foreseeable or preventable discomforts or risks for the researcher and/or the study population.

The research data was collected and analysed by the researcher alone, with the intention of protecting the documents studied. Confidential and sensitive information was not analysed. The name or any other means of identifying the patient in the study was not used. The data collected from the patients will be anonymised.

This study was submitted to the Research Ethics Committee of Unicamp's Faculty of Medical Sciences and approved under number 308/2008 (CAEE 0240.0.146.000-080).

CHAPTER 5

RESULTS

5.1- Profile of the rural workers studied

Most of the patients studied were aged between 35 and 39.

Table 1- Distribution of the patients studied according to age

Age (years)	Absolute frequency	Relative percentage	Cumulative relative percentage
Below 20	17	5,0	5,0
From the 20th to the 24th	41	11,0	16,0
From the 25th to the 29th	40	10,8	26,8
From 30 to 34	45	12,1	38,9
From 35 to 39	56	15,1	54,0
From 40 to 44	48	13,0	67,0
From 45 to 49	34	9,1	76,1
From 50 to 54	38	10,2	86,3
From 55 to 59	30	8,1	94,4
From 60	21	5,6	100,0
Total	**370**	*100,0*	

The predominant gender was male, corresponding to 71.35 per cent of the sample studied.

Table 2- Distribution of patients according to gender

Sex	Absolute frequency	Relative percentage
Female	106	28,65
Male	264	71,35
Total	**370**	**100**

With regard to the use of alcoholic beverages, 33.24% of the patients studied were considered to be alcoholics (alcohol consumption above 20g alcohol/week), as shown in Table 3:

Table 3- Distribution of patients according to alcohol consumption

Alcoholism	Absolute frequency	Relative percentage
No	247	66,76
Yes	123	33,24
Total	**370**	**100**

With regard to metabolic alterations, these were present in 8.11% of the patients studied, according to Table 4

Table 4- Distribution of patients according to the presence of metabolic alterations

Metabolic change	Absolute frequency	Relative percentage
No	340	91,89
Yes	30	8,11
Total	*370*	*100*

Among the labour relations studied, 48.92% of the workers reported being wage earners, 25.14% sharecroppers, 19.73% owners, 4.86% had other employment relationships and

1.35% were free-lance workers.

Table 5- Distribution of patients according to work relationship

Working relationship	Absolute frequency	Relative percentage
Salaried	181	48,92
Steward	93	25,14
Owner	73	19,73
Steering wheel	4	1,35
Other	18	4,86
Total	*370*	*100*

With regard to the type of exposure workers had to pesticides, two types of contact were defined. Direct contact was when the farmer applied, prepared and diluted the pesticide and when he washed the clothes used in the application. And indirect contact was related to planting, harvesting, weeding, packaging, pruning and weeding.

According to Table 6, the majority of workers had direct contact with pesticides (85.14 per cent).

Table 6- Distribution of patients according to type of contact with pesticides

Type of contact	Absolute frequency	Relative percentage
Direct	315	85,14
Indirect	55	14,6
Total	**370**	**100**

With regard to the use of PPE (personal protective equipment), 78.65 per cent reported using it. The rest did not report using any type of PPE.

The PPE surveyed included wearing long trousers, a long-sleeved shirt, suitable waterproof clothing, closed shoes, boots, gloves, goggles, masks, hats or caps.

Table 7- Distribution of patients according to the use of PPE

Use of PPE	Absolute frequency	Relative percentage
No	79	21,35
Yes	291	78,65
Total	**370**	**100**

With regard to how the workers arrived at the HC-Unicamp Toxicology Outpatient Clinic, it was found that the majority (85.68%) were the result of an active search, which consists of fieldwork carried out by the Toxicology and Environmental Health discipline of the Department of Preventive and Social Medicine (DMPS) of the Faculty of Medical Sciences (FCM) at Unicamp. In this work, students together with lecturers assess various rural communities in the Campinas-SP region and refer patients with symptoms or a history of hospitalisation for pesticide poisoning or laboratory alterations to be assessed at the outpatient clinic.

The other referrals came 3.78% from the Unicamp JRC, 8.11% from regional health centres, 0.27% from the CRST (Workers' Health Reference Centre) and 2.16% from other specialities that provide outpatient care at HC-Unicamp, as shown in Table 8:

Table 8- Distribution of patients according to type of referral

Type of referral	Absolute frequency	Relative percentage
Active Search	317	85,68
CCI Unicamp	14	3,78
Health centres	30	8,11
CRST	1	0,27
Other specialities	8	2,16
Total	**370**	**100**

Analysing Table 9, it can be concluded that 45.94% of the workers studied had been exposed to more than one chemical group of pesticides, as described above, which was called combined exposure.

Table 9- Distribution of patients according to combined exposure

Exhibition	Absolute frequency	Relative percentage
No	105	28,38
Yes	170	45,94
Don't know	95	25,68
Total	**370**	**100**

4.3- Analysis of the alterations found in the physical and laboratory examinations and the diagnoses made

According to Table 10, alterations in the patients' physical examination were present in 16.22% of them:

Table 10- Distribution of patients according to physical alteration

Physical change	Absolute frequency	Relative percentage
No	310	83,78
Yes	60	16,22
Total	**370**	**100**

Among the alterations in the physical examination, dermatological alterations were the most frequent, with 32% of the alterations, followed by alterations in the peripheral neurological examination, present in 16.7% of the patients who presented alterations in the physical examination.

The dermatological alterations found were characterised as: irritant and sensitivity contact dermatitis, solar melanosis and pityriasis versicolor. The peripheral neurological examination revealed decreased muscle strength, paresthesia and decreased tactile and painful sensitivity in the lower limbs.

Ophthalmological alterations were present in 13.3 per cent of patients, abdominal alterations in 10 per cent and, lastly, respiratory system alterations in 6.7 per cent of patients, as shown in Table 11.

Among the alterations found in the ophthalmological examination were pterygium and red eye syndromes. In the abdominal examination the alterations found were characterised as hepatomegaly and splenomegaly and in the respiratory examination the signs of bronchial hyperreactivity syndromes were present.

Table 11- Distribution of patients according to the type of alteration on physical examination.

Type of change	Absolute frequency	Relative percentage
Abdominal examination	6	10,0
Dermatological examination	32	53,3
Respiratory examination	4	6,7
Neurological examination	10	16,7
Ophthalmological examination	8	13,3
Total	**60**	**100**

Laboratory alterations were found in 29.73% of the patients studied, as shown in Table 12:

Table 12- Distribution of patients according to laboratory alterations

Laboratory changes	Absolute frequency	Relative percentage
No	260	70,27
Yes	110	29,73
Total	**370**	**100**

According to the table below, 37.21 per cent of the patients with alterations in the laboratory test had alterations in the cholinesterase test using the Elman method:

Table 13- Distribution of patients according to cholinesterase alterations.

Alteration of cholinesterase	Absolute frequency	Relative percentage
No	69	62,8
Yes	41	37,2
Total	**110**	**100**

Of the changes in cholinesterase, 78 per cent were due to changes in plasma cholinesterase and only 22 per cent to changes in erythrocyte cholinesterase, as shown in Table 14:

Table 14- Distribution of patients according to the type of cholinesterase alteration

Changes in cholinesterase	Absolute frequency	Relative percentage
Plasma cholinesterase	32	78
Erythrocyte cholinesterase	9	22
Total	**41**	**100**

Among the patients with laboratory alterations, 26.3% had haematological alterations, most of which (41.4%) were due to thrombocytopenia, 34.5% to neutropenia, 20.6% to anaemia and 3.5% to pancytopenia (Tables 15 and 16).

Table 15- Distribution of patients according to haematological alteration

Amendment	Absolute frequency	Relative percentage
No	81	73,7
Yes	29	26,3

Total	110	100

Table 16- Distribution of types of haematological alteration

Type of change	Absolute frequency	Relative percentage
Anaemia	6	20,6
Thrombocytopenia	12	41,4
Pancytopenia	1	3,5
Neutropenia	10	34,5
Total	29	100

As for liver alterations, they were found in 37.2% of patients with alterations in laboratory tests, and the majority had altered GGT (35.6%), followed by altered AST (31.6%), ALT (28.9%) and finally F.A (3.9%), as shown in Tables 17 and 18:

Table 17- Distribution of patients according to liver alterations

Amendment	Absolute frequency	Relative percentage
No	69	62,8
Yes	41	37,2
Total	110	100

Table 18- Distribution of types of liver alteration

Type of change	Absolute frequency	Relative percentage
ALT	22	28,9
AST	24	31,6
GGT	27	35,6
FA	3	3,9
Total	76	100

Of the 41 patients with hepatic alterations, 9, or 21.9%, had some kind of metabolic alteration, as shown in Table 19:

Table 19- Association between metabolic alteration and hepatic alteration

Metabolic change	Altered liver profile		
	No	Yes	Total
No	48	32	80
Yes	21	9	30
Total	69	41	110

p = 0.002 (Fisher's exact test)

Of the 41 patients with liver disorders, 22, or 53.6%, were alcoholics, as shown in Table 20:

Table 20- Association between alcoholism and liver changes

Alcoholism	Altered liver profile		
	No	Yes	Total
No	44	19	63
Yes	25	22	47
Total	69	41	110

p = 0.074 (Fisher's exact test)

Among the patients with laboratory alterations, 21.8% had renal alterations, according to Table 21:

Table 21- Distribution of patients according to renal alteration

Amendment	Absolute frequency	Relative percentage
No	86	78,2
Yes	24	21,8
Total	**110**	**100**

Of the kidney changes, 73.7% were due to alterations in the MICROALB and 26.3% change in A1M (Table 22):

Table 22- Distribution of types of renal alteration.

Type of change	Absolute frequency	Relative percentage
MICROALB	19	73,7
A1M	5	26,3
Total	**24**	**100**

Among the 24 patients with renal alterations, 3 (12.5%) presented some kind of metabolic alteration, as shown in Table 23:

Table 23- Association between metabolic alteration and renal alteration

Metabolic change	Altered renal profile		
	No	Yes	Total
No	59	21	80
Yes	27	3	30
Total	**86**	**24**	**110**

p = 0.99 (Fisher's exact test)

With regard to the diagnoses established for the patients studied, these were: "Long-term exposure to pesticides" when the patients assessed did not show any alterations in their physical or laboratory tests, and "Health effects" when these patients showed any alterations in their physical and/or laboratory tests that could be considered harmful to their health.

According to Table 24, the majority of patients, i.e. 79.2 per cent, were diagnosed with long-term exposure to pesticides and only 20.8 per cent were diagnosed with "health effects":

Table 24- Distribution of patients according to type of diagnosis

Diagnosis	Absolute frequency	Relative percentage
Health effects	77	20,8
Long-term exposure to pesticides	293	79,2
Total	**370**	**100**

4.4- Association between demographic variables, habits and work-related aspects and alterations in physical examination, laboratory tests and diagnosis

Analysing the effect of each variable studied (gender, age, alcohol consumption, presence of metabolic alterations, type of referral, work relationship, type of contact, use of PPE and combined exposure) on the chance of having alterations in the physical examination, there was no evidence to conclude a significant association between any of these variables and alterations in the physical examination (p>0.05 chi-squared test), as shown in Table 25:

Table 25- Comparison between workers with and without alterations in the physical examination in relation to demographic, habit, service and labour characteristics, HC - Unicamp, 2006 and 2007

Features	Changes on physical examination		P	OR[5]	CI(OR;95%)
	No (n = 310)	Yes (n = 60)			
Sex			0,1051		
Female	30,3%	20,0%		1,00	
Male	69,7%	80,0%		1,74	(0,88 - 3,42)
Age (years)	38,0(27,0 ; 48,0)	40,0(33,0 ; 51,7)	0,050[2]		
Alcoholic			0,987[1]		
No	66,8%	66,7%		1,00	
Yes	33,2%	33,3%		1,005	(0,55 - 1,80)
Metabolic change			0,270[1]		
No	92,6%	88,3%		1,00	
Yes	7,4%	11,7%		1,64	(0,67 - 4,03)
Type of referral			0,407[3]		
Active search	86,5%	81,7%		1,00	
CCI Unicamp	3,5%	5,0%		1,49	(0,40 - 5,54)
Health centre	8,1%	8,3%		1,09	(0,40 - 3,00)
CRST	0,3%	0,0%		---	---
Other specialities	1,6%	5,0%		3,28	(0,76 - 14,18)
Working relationship			0,698[3]		
Owner	20,0%	18,3%		1,00	
Steward	23,9%	31,7%		1,45	(0,64 - 3,27)
Diarist	0,3%	0,0%		---	---
Steering wheel	1,0%	1,7%		1,88	(0,18 - 19,75)
Salaried	49,7%	45,0%		0,99	(0,46 - 2,11)
Other	5,2%	3,3%		0,70	(0,14 - 3,50)
Type of contact			0,447[1]		
Indirect	15,5%	11,7%		1,00	
Direct	84,5%	88,3%		1,38	(0,59 - 3,23)
Use of PPE			0,682[1]		
Yes	79,0%	76,7%			
No	21,0%	23,3%		1,14	(0,59 - 2,21)
Combined exposure	(n = 224)[4]	(n = 51)[4]	0,880[1]		
No	38,4%	37,3%		1,00	
Yes	61,6%	62,7%		1,05	(0,56 - 1,96)

(1) Chi-squared test.

(2) Mann-Whitney test. Descriptive summary in median and quartiles.

(3) Fisher's exact test.

(4) Number of patients who could answer about combined exposure

(5) Odds-Ratio estimate.

Table 26 shows a significant association between alcohol consumption and alterations in laboratory tests (p-value of 0.012 Chi-square test).

Table 26- Comparison between workers with and without laboratory test alterations in relation to demographic, habit, service and labour characteristics, HC - Unicamp, 2006 and 2007

Features	Change by No (n = 260)	laboratory test Yes (n = 110)	P	OR[5]	CI(OR;95%)
Sex			0,377[1]		
Female	30,0%	25,5%		1,00	
Male	70,0%	74,5%		1,25	(0,75 - 2,07)
Age (years)	38,0(29,0 ;49,0)	39,5(29,0 ;49,2)	0,483[2]		
Alcoholic			0,012[1]		
No	70,8%	57,3%		1,00	
Yes	29,2%	42,7%		1,80	(1,13 - 2,86)
Metabolic change			0,386[1]		
No	92,7%	90,0%		1,00	
Yes	7,3%	10,0%		1,40	(0,64 - 3,07)
Type of referral			0,084[3]		
Active search	85,8%	85,5%		1,00	
CCI Unicamp	3,1%	5,5%		1,78	(0,60 - 5,27)

	9,6%	4,5%		0,47	(0,18 - 1,28)
Health centre	9,6%	4,5%		0,47	(0,18 - 1,28)
CRST	0,0%	0,9%		---	---
Other specialities	1,5%	3,6%		2,37	(0,58 - 9,69)
Working relationship			0,864[3]		
Owner	20,0%	19,1%		1,00	
Steward	25,0%	25,5%		1,07	(0,54 - 2,09)
Diarist	0,4%	0,0%		---	---
Steering wheel	1,2%	0,9%		0,83	(0,08 - 8,39)
Salaried	47,7%	51,8%		1,14	(0,63 - 2,07)
Other	5,8%	2,7%		0,50	(0,13 - 1,89)
Type of contact			0,452[1]		
Indirect	15,8%	12,7%		1,00	
Direct	84,2%	87,3%		1,28	(0,66 - 2,46)
Use of PPE			0,128[1]		
Yes	76,5%	83,6%		1,00	
No	23,5%	16,4%		0,63	(0,35 - 1,14)
Combined exposure	(n = 192)[4]	(n = 83)[4]	0,205[1]		
No	40,6%	32,5%		1,00	
Yes	59,4%	67,5%		1,41	(0,82 - 2,44)

(1) Chi-squared test.

(2) Mann-Whitney test. Descriptive summary in median and quartiles.

(3) Fisher's exact test.

(4) Number of patients who could answer about combined exposure

(5) Odds-Ratio estimate.

Table 27 shows a significant association between age, alcohol consumption and metabolic alterations in relation to the diagnosis "Health effects", all with p-values < 0.05 using the Chi-square test. The use of PPE was not considered to have a significant association, since the confidence interval for this association is between 0.23 and 0.99, and thus the upper limit practically encompasses 1, making it impossible to categorically state that there was a significant effect.

Table 27- Comparison between workers without and with health effects detected by diagnosis in relation to demographic, habit, service and labour characteristics, HC - Unicamp, 2006 and 2007

	Diagnosis				
Features	Long-term exposure to pesticides (n = 293)	Other health effects (n = 77)	p	OR[5]	CI(OR;95%)
Sex			0,086[1]		
Female	30,7%	20,8%		1,00	
Male	69,3%	79,2%		1,69	(0,92 - 3,09)
Age (years)	38,0(27,0 ; 47,0)	43,0(34,5 ; 52,5)	0,001[2]		
Alcoholic			0,022[1]		
No	69,6%	55,8%		1,00	
Yes	30,4%	44,2%		1,81	(1,08 - 3,03)
Metabolic change			0,026[1]		
No	93,5%	85,7%		1,00	
Yes	6,5%	14,3%		2,40	(1,09 - 5,29)
Type of referral			0,111[3]		
Active search	85,7%	85,7%		1,00	
CCI Unicamp	3,4%	5,2%		1,52	(0,46 - 5,00)
Health centre	9,2%	3,9%		0,42	(0,12 - 1,44)
CRST	0,3%	0,0%		---	---
Other specialities	1,4%	5,2%		3,80	(0,93 - 15,61)
Working relationship			0,099[3]		
Owner	18,1%	26,0%		1,00	
Steward	24,6%	27,3%		0,77	(0,38 - 1,57)
Diarist	0,3%	0,0%		---	---
Steering wheel	1,4%	0,0%		---	---
Salaried	49,5%	46,8%		0,66	(0,35 - 1,24)
Other	6,1%	0,0%		---	---
Type of contact			0,603[1]		
Indirect	15,4%	13,0%		1,00	
Direct	84,6%	87,0%		1,21	(0,58 - 2,53)

Use of PPE			*0,044*[3]		
Yes	76,5%	87,0%		1,00	
No	23,5%	13,0%		0,48	(0,23 - 0,99)
Combined exposure	(n = 215)[4]	(n = 60)[4]	*0,382*[3]		
No	39,5%	33,3%		1,00	
Yes	60,5%	66,7%		1,30	(0,71 - 2,38)

(1) Chi-squared test

(2) Mann-Whitney test. Descriptive summary in median and quartiles.

(3) Fisher's exact test.

(4) Number of patients who could answer about combined exposure

(5) Odds-Ratio estimation.

5.4- Study of the Effect of Time of Exposure to Pesticides on the Occurrence of Changes in Physical and Laboratory Examination and Diagnosis

5.4.1- Study of the effect of exposure time to pesticides on changes in health status by physical examination.

According to Table 25, the worker's age was the characteristic that had the greatest effect on the change in health status by physical examination (p=0.05; Mann-Whitney test). However, Graph 2 shows that both groups have a similar range and distribution of ages

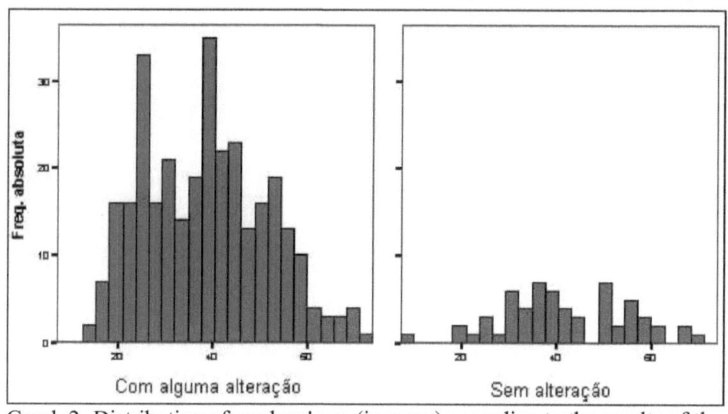

Graph 2- Distribution of workers' age (in years) according to the results of the physical examination

According to Table 28, the workers who showed some alteration in the physical examination were statistically exposed to pesticides for a longer period of time than the workers who did not show any alteration in the physical examination.

Table 28- Comparison between patients with and without any alterations on physical examination in relation to time of exposure to pesticides, HC-Unicamp, 2006 and 2007

	Changes on physical examination				
	No	Yes	P	OR[2]	CI(95%;OR)
Exposure time (years)	10,0(4,0 ; 20,0)	16,0(7,2 ; 26,0)	0,029[1]	1,02	(1,003 - 1,046)

(1) Mann-Whitney test for independent samples. Descriptive summary in median and quartiles.

(2) Point estimate of the Odds-Ratio.

    5.4.2- Study of the effect of exposure time to pesticides on changes in health status by laboratory examination

According to Table 26, 29 per cent of the workers with no alterations in the laboratory test declared that they were alcoholics, while 42.7 per cent of the workers with alterations in the laboratory test were alcoholics. Recognising the limitations of the information in the medical records and assuming that the amount of alcohol ingested is similar among alcoholics with and without alterations, it can be concluded that there was a significant association between alcoholism and alterations in the laboratory test (p=0.012; Chi-squared test).

Furthermore, according to Table 29, 50 per cent of non-alcoholics had been exposed to pesticides for less than ten years, while among alcoholics, 50 per cent had been exposed for more than fifteen years (p= 0.047; Mann-Whitney test).

Graph 3 shows that the distribution of exposure times among non-drinkers is more concentrated among the shorter exposure times. Therefore, the study of the effect of exposure time on the occurrence of alterations in the laboratory test was carried out by isolating the effect of alcohol consumption, as shown in Table 30.

Table 29- Comparison between alcoholics and non-alcoholics in relation to exposure time to pesticides

	Alcoholic		p
	No (n=247)	Yes (n=123)	
Exposure time (years)	10,0 (4,0 ; 20,0)	15,0 (6,0 ; 25,0)	0.047)(1

(1) Mann-Whitney test for independent samples. Descriptive summary in median and quartiles.

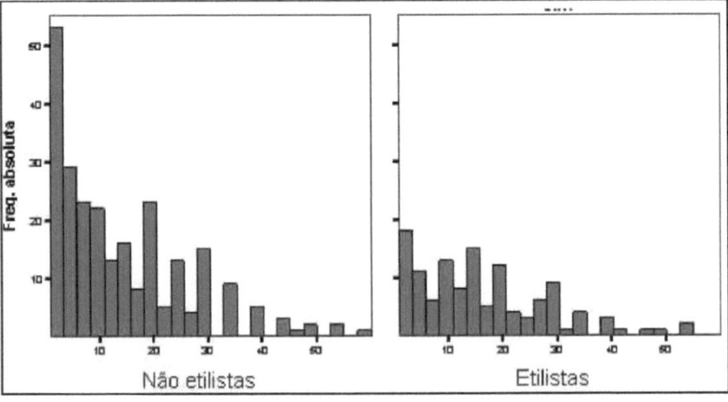

Graph 3- Distribution of exposure time to pesticides (in years) among alcoholic and non-alcoholic workers, HC-Unicamp, 2006 and 2007

Table 30- Median and quartiles of time exposed to pesticides, HC-Unicamp, 2006 and 2007

| | Change in laboratory test | | $p^{(1)}$ | $OR^{(2)}$ | CI(OR;95%) |
	No	Yes			
Non-drinkers	10,0(4,0 ; 20,0) (n = 184)	10,0(4,0 ; 20,0) (n = 63)	0,999	0,99	(0,97 -1,02)
Alcoholics	14,0(5,0 ; 22,7) (n=76)	15,0(10,0 ; 25,0) (n=47)	0,308	1,01	(0,98 - 1,04)

(1) Mann-Whitney test for independent samples.

(2) Point estimate of the Odds-Ratio.

As Table 30 illustrates, there was no significant difference between workers with and without alterations in the laboratory test in relation to time of exposure to pesticides, regardless of alcohol consumption.

5.4.3- Study of the effect of exposure time to pesticides on diagnosis

Graph 4 shows a positive correlation between worker age and exposure time, i.e. older workers have been exposed to pesticides for longer and, according to Spearman's correlation coefficient, this correlation was significant ($r = 0.616$; $p < 0.01$).

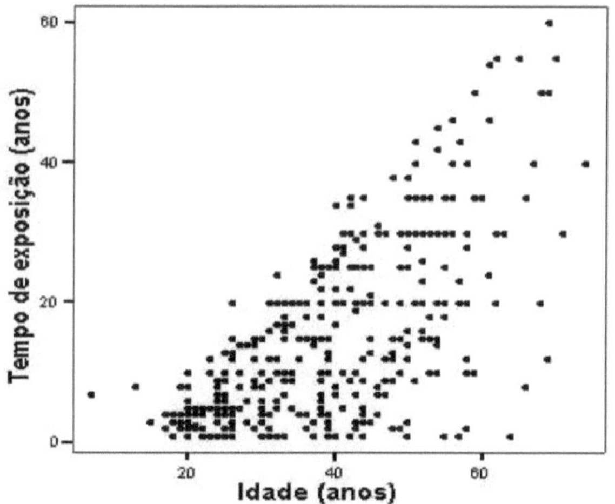

Graph 4 - Scatter plot between age and length of exposure of workers to pesticides, HC-Unicamp, 2006 and 2007.

Table 31- Comparison between workers with and without metabolic alterations in relation to time of exposure to pesticides, HC-Unicamp, 2006 and 2007

| | Metabolic change | | p |
	No (n=340)	Yes(n=30)	
Exposure time (years)	12,0 (4,0 ; 21,5)	15,0 (7,0 ; 26,5)	0,111(1)

(1) Mann-Whitney test for independent samples. Descriptive summary in median and quartiles.

Table 32- Comparison between workers who used and did not use PPE in relation to time of exposure to pesticides, HC-Unicamp, 2006 and 2007

| | Used PPE | | p |
	No (n=291)	Yes (n=79)	
Exposure time (years)	13,0 (5,0 ; 23,0)	10,0 (3,0 ; 20,0)	0,061()

(1) Mann-Whitney test for independent samples. Descriptive summary in median and quartiles.

According to Graph 4 and Tables 29, 31 and 32, the study of the effect of exposure time to pesticides on diagnosis will be carried out taking into account the effects of alcohol consumption and age

Table 33- Adjusted logistic model to explain the diagnosis of Health Effects as a function of age and time of exposure to pesticides among alcoholics and non-alcoholics, HC-Unicamp, 2006 and 2007

Alcoholism		Estimate of β	P	OR	IC(OR;95%
	Age	0,05	0,034	1,05	(1,00 - 1,09)
	Exposure time	0,07	0,223	1,08	(0,96 - 1,21)
No	Age x Exposure time	0,00	0,169	1,00	(0,99 - 1,00)
	Intercept	-3,40	0,000	0,03	
	x_2= 5.46 ; gl = 3 ; p = 0.140				
	Age	0,06	0,047	1,06	(1,00 - 1,12)
	Exposure time	0,06	0,374	1,07	(0,93 - 1,23)
Yes	Age x Exposure time	0,00	0,388	1,00	(0,99 - 1,00)
	Intercept	-3,54	0,004	0,03	
	x_2= 7.66 ; gl = 3 ; p = 0.054				

According to the logistic model in Table 33, there was no effect of time on the diagnosis of "Health effects".

CHAPTER 6

DISCUSSION

Analysing the results obtained on the profile of rural workers, it was found that the majority of patients were aged between 35 and 39 and 71.35% were male. This was to be expected, as many studies have shown similar results, such as Soares (2005), Faria et al.(2004) and Moreira et al.(2002).

Among the labour relations found, the majority of the workers studied, i.e. almost half (48.92%), are salaried, showing that employment in rural areas is still widespread and that rural workers depend on the attitudes and decisions of their bosses.

With regard to contact with pesticides, the majority (85.14%) had direct contact, showing that pesticides are still handled a lot, but in a protected manner, as 78.65% of patients reported using personal protective equipment (PPE).

Regarding the way in which workers arrived at the Toxicology Outpatient Centre, it was found that the majority, 85.68%, came from active searches, which demonstrates the need to carry out field work and to seek out rural workers at their place of work, as this can demonstrate both difficulty in accessing health services and a lack of information among rural workers about the damage that pesticides can cause to their health.

Table 9 shows that most of the workers (45.94%) had combined exposure to all the pesticide groups, demonstrating that the symptoms presented by the patients may be associated with the combined effects of these pesticides. However, one fact that drew attention was that 25.68% of the patients studied did not know the type of pesticide they were using, demonstrating that they are not the ones who prepare the product or reinforcing the studies by Tomazin (2007) and Oliveira et al. (2001) which showed that the majority of rural workers do not read pesticide leaflets and labels.

With regard to the alterations found during the physical examination, it can be seen that the majority of patients did not have any, i.e. 83.78%. Of those who did, most were dermatological (53.3%), most likely due to sun exposure (solar melanosis) and unprotected contact with pesticides (contact dermatitis).

Laboratory alterations were present in 29.73% of the patients studied, and the predominant alteration was the liver profile, corresponding to 37.2% of the alterations found. However, an analysis of Tables 18 and 20 showed that 35.6% of liver alterations were due to GGT and that more than half of the patients with liver alterations (53.6%) were alcoholics, which confirms that alcoholism is an important risk factor for the liver alterations found. With regard to the association between metabolic alterations and alterations in the liver profile, Table 19 shows that only 21.9% of the patients with liver alterations had some metabolic disorder, which is a risk factor that had a lesser influence on the genesis of these alterations in the patients studied, when compared to alcoholism.

With regard to cholinesterase alterations, it was found that 37.21% of the patients with alterations in the laboratory test had alterations in the cholinesterase dosage test using the Elman method, and that the majority of these alterations were due to plasma cholinesterase (78%) and only 22% due to erythrocyte cholinesterase. It is known that alterations in plasma cholinesterase can be due to hepatic alterations, because this enzyme is produced in this organ, due to the use of certain drugs with hepatic metabolisation and can also be idiopathic. Therefore, this information alone does not allow us to characterise these patients as intoxicated. With regard to the nine patients who had altered erythrocyte cholinesterase levels, they were taken off work and monitored. After three months, their erythrocyte cholinesterase levels normalised, which may suggest that the alteration was due to exposure to cholinesterase-inhibiting pesticides. However, this data does not mean that the patients who had a change in erythrocyte cholinesterase were intoxicated, since these patients did not show any changes in the physical examination or other laboratory alterations.

Among the haematological alterations found, they were present in 29% of the patients who presented laboratory alterations, the majority of which were due to thrombocytopenia (41.4%), followed by neutropenia (34.5%), then anaemia (20.6%) and finally pancytopenia (3.5%). These alterations may be related to the presence of solvents in pesticide formulations.

Renal alterations were the least common, with 21.8% of patients showing alterations in laboratory tests, most of which were due to alterations in microalbuminuria (73.7%) and 26.3% to alterations in alpha 1 microglobulin. Among the patients who presented renal alterations, 12.5% had some metabolic alteration, which may partly explain these changes.

In this sense, a more detailed analysis of the laboratory alterations found, relating them to the diagnoses made, shows in Table 24 that the majority of patients, i.e. 79.2 per cent, were diagnosed with long-term exposure to pesticides and 20.8 per cent with the diagnosis of health effects, demonstrating that even with long-term exposure to pesticides, the majority of workers did not develop significant damage to their health.

When analysing the associations between the variables studied and alterations in the physical examination, laboratory tests and diagnosis, it was found that the physical examination was not influenced by any of the variables studied, with age being the characteristic that came closest to having an influence. With regard to laboratory tests, alcohol consumption showed a significant association. With regard to diagnosis, alcohol consumption, metabolic alterations and age showed a significant association, which is somewhat understandable, given that older people are more likely to have alterations in their state of health and alcohol and metabolic alterations are risk factors for a large number of comorbidities.

With regard to the effect of time on alterations in the physical examination, laboratory tests and diagnosis, it was found that the workers who presented any alterations in the physical examination had been exposed to pesticides for a longer period of time. This may show that patients who started using pesticides less recently are showing fewer health effects than those who have been exposed for longer. This may be due to the use of personal protective equipment, which is now more widely available and used by rural workers. Laboratory changes and diagnosis were not influenced by time.

CHAPTER 7

CONCLUSION

This study, carried out with 370 patients seen at Unicamp's Toxicology Outpatient Clinic in 2006 and 2007, concluded that:

- Most of the patients studied were male and aged between 35 and 39.

- The main way patients came to the Toxicology Outpatient Clinic was through active search.

- Most of the patients had direct contact with pesticides.

- Most of the patients studied reported using personal protective equipment.

- The vast majority of patients who were exposed to pesticides over the long term did not show any significant changes in their state of health.

- The physical examination alone was not enough to suspect any damage to the patient's health.

- Among the laboratory tests assessed, the liver profile was the one that showed the most alterations, but in 53.6% of the patients with liver alterations, alcoholism was present.

- Alcohol consumption was the characteristic that most influenced the search for laboratory alterations and the diagnosis.

- The most prevalent diagnosis in the patients studied was long-term exposure to pesticides.

CHAPTER 8

FINAL CONSIDERATIONS

Although the use of pesticides is associated with serious environmental and especially public health impacts, with reports of contamination of the various media (air, water and soil), and cases of acute poisoning and death, this study did not show that the long-term use of these substances causes major health effects for workers.

Nowadays, many factors contribute to the effects of long-term exposure to pesticides not being so devastating to health. Today's rural workers have more information about pesticides, more access to personal protective equipment (PPE) and more modern application technologies, and better hygiene and working conditions, which was not the case 20 years ago, partly due to the current greater supervision of working environments.

The health alterations investigated in the patients in this study were within the scope of Clinical Toxicology, assessing the patients through complaints, physical examination and the markers of exposure and effects currently described in the literature. In all likelihood, the methods used in this study could be surpassed in the future with the discovery of new markers of exposure and effects on the health of patients exposed to pesticides and/or by molecular toxicology studies.

CHAPTER 9

REFERENCES Almeida, WF. Accidental human poisoning by insecticides. O Biológico, 2.ed. Publication no. 120, 1967.

Almeida, WF. Agricultural labour and its relationship with ill health. In: Mendes, R. Pathologia do Trabalho. São Paulo: Atheneu, 1995. p. 487-544.

Alonzo HGA, Correa CL. Pesticides. In:Oga S. Fundamentos de Toxicologia, 2.ed. São Paulo: Atheneu; 2003: 339-458.

Alonzo HGA. Acute poisoning by pesticides in the toxicology centres of six university hospitals in Brazil in 1994 [Master's thesis]. Campinas (SP): State University of Campinas; 1995.

Alonzo HGA. Consultation in Six Poison Control Centres in Brazil: Analysis of Cases, Hospitalisations and Deaths. Campinas, 2000 (Doctoral Thesis - State University of Campinas).

Araújo ACP, Augusto LGS, Telles DL. The issue of pesticides in agriculture and the situation in the state of Pernambuco. Rev. Brasileira de Toxicologia 2000a; 13(1): 25-30.

National Plant Defence Association. ANDEF. Andef presents profile of the crop protection sector to Conab executives. Available at: http://www.andef.com.br/2008/noticias.asp/numero=602. Accessed on: 05/11/2008.

Brazil, 1997. Ministry of Health. Health Surveillance Secretariat. Health Surveillance Manual for Populations Exposed to Pesticides. Pan American Health Organisation/World Health Organisation. Brasilia.

Bull, D & Hathaway, D. Pragas e venenos: agrotóxicos no Brasil e no terceiro mundo. Petrópolis - R.J, Vozes/Oxafam/Fase, 1986.23p.

Chediack, R 1986. Occupational health in the field of agrochemicals, PP. 119139. In Pan American Centre for Ecology and Health Pan American Health Organisation 9orgs.) Plaguicida, salud y ambiente: memórias de los tallers de san cristóbal de las Casas. Chiapas, Mexico.

Council On Scientific Affairs. Education and Information strategies to reduce pesticide risks. Preventive Medicine 1997; 26: 191-200.

Echobicon DJ. Toxic effects of peticides. In: Amdur, M.O; Doull,J; klassen, C.D. ed. *Casarett and Doull's Toxicology: The basic science of poisons. 4* ed. McGraW-Hill INC, New York, 1993. p 566-622.

Ellenhorn, MJ & Barceloux, DG. Pesticides. In: Medical toxicology: diagnosis and treatment of human poisoning. New York, Elsevier, 1988.p 1067-1108.

Faria , NMX; FachiniI LA; Fassa AG; Tomasin E.Rural Labour and Poisoning by Pesticides. Cad. Saúde Pública 2004: 20 (5): 1298-1308.

Fernandes,G. General classification of plaguicides. In: Intoxication by plaguicides: physiopathology, clinic and treatment. Montevideo, 1970. p. 35-46.

Freitas CU *et al.* 1986. Epidemiological Surveillance Project in the Ribeira Valley. Occupational Health and Safety Journal 21(3):107-118

Gallo MA. History and Scope of Toxicology. In: Casarett and Doull's Toxicology: the basic science of poisons, 5ª edition, 1996, pg 3-11.

Garcia EG 1996. Safety and Health in rural work with pesticides: a contribution to a more comprehensive approach. Master's thesis. School of Public Health, University of São Paulo, São Paulo.

Garcia, E & ALMEIDA, WF. Exposure of rural workers to pesticides in Brazil. Rev Bras Saúde Ocup, 19: 7-11, 1991.

Garcia,E. Safety and Health in Rural Labour: The Question of Pesticides. São Paulo: Fundacentro, 2001.

IBGE - Brazilian Institute of Geography and Statistics. Population count estimates 2007. Available at http://www.ibge.gov.br. Accessed on: 15/11/2008.

Kaloyanova, F. Interaction of pesticides. In:Health effects of combined exposure to chemicals in work and communities environments. Copenhagen, WHO Regional Office for Europe, p.165 -195 (Interim document 11), 1983.

Kotaka ET. Contributions to the construction of toxicological risk assessment guidelines for pesticides [Dissertation]. Campinas (SP): State University of Campinas; 2000.

Meirelles, LC 1996. Control of pesticides: a case study of the state of Rio de Janeiro, 1985/1995. [Dissertation]. Postgraduate Engineering Programme, Federal University of Rio de Janeiro, Rio de Janeiro.

Moreira JC et al. 2002. Integrated assessment of the impact of pesticide use on human health in an agricultural community in Nova Friburgo, RJ. Ciência e Saúde Coletiva 7(2):299-311.

Morris, B; BLAIR,A; Gilsson R; Everetti, G; Cantor, K; Schuman, L et al. Pesticides exposures and agricultural risk factors for leukemia among men in Iowa and Minnesota. Cancer. Res. 1998; 50: 6585 - 6591.

Nishiyama, P. Utilização de agrotóxicos em áreas de reforma agrária no estado do Paraná [Tese-Doutorado]. Campinas (S.P): State University of Campinas; 2003.

ILO 2001. Agriculture and sectors based on biological resources, pp. 64.2-64.77. In Enciclopedia de Salud y Seguridad en el Trabajo, vol. III, part X, chapter 64. *Available at http://www.mtas.es/Publica/enciclo/default.htm.Acesso on: 05/04/2008.*

Oliveira JJS; Alves SR; Peres F, Sarcinelli PN; Mattos RCOC; Moreira JC.Influence of Socioeconomic Factors on Pesticide Contamination. Brazil. Rev. Saúde Pública 2001; 35 (2): 130-35.

Oliveira MLF. Vulnerability and care in the use of pesticides by family farmers [PhD Thesis]. Campinas (SP): State University of Campinas; 2004.

Peres F. Is it poison or is it medicine? The challenges of rural communication about pesticides [Dissertation]. Rio de Janeiro (RJ): Oswaldo Cruz Foundation - National School of Public Health; 1999.

Peres F, Rozemberg B, Alves SR, Moreira, JC & Oliveira-Silva JJ 2001. Communication related to the use of pesticides in an agricultural region of the State of Rio de Janeiro. Revista de Saúde Pública 35(6):564-570.

Planet, N. Poisoning produced by insecticides in rural workers fighting cotton pests. Rev. Paul . Méd., 37: 59-60,1950.

Plimmer, JR. Chemistry of pesticides. In: Krieger, RI. Handbook of pesticide toxicology, 2ª edition, Academic Press, 2001. p. 95-107

Rodrigues, D.C; Planet, N; Ginnotti, O. Intoxications by insecticides. O Biológico, 1957.

Rosenstokl. et al. Chronic central nervous system effects of acute organophosphate pesticide intoxication. The Lancet, 338: 223-226, 1991.

Sauad, J 1984. Rural Credit in Brazil. Ed. FIPE/Pioneira, São Paulo.

Paraná State Health Department1983... Epidemiological Surveillance Programme in Pesticide Ecotoxicology. Mimeo,

Silva, A.A. Late Evaluation of the Health Status of People Acutely Poisoned by Cholinesterase Inhibiting Pesticides. Campinas: 2004 (PhD Thesis - State University of Campinas).

SINITOX - National Toxic-Pharmacological Information System. Registered Cases of Human Intoxication and Poisoning. Brazil, 2006. Available at: http://www.fiocruz.br/sinitox/. Accessed on: 22/11/2008.

Siqueira, M.L; Jacob, A; Canhete, R.L. Diagnosis of Ecotoxicological Problems Caused by the Use of Agricultural Defensives in the State of Paraná. Rev . Brás. Saúde Ocupacional, 11 (44): 7-17, 1983.

Soares, WL; Freitas EAV; Coutinho JAG. Rural labour and health: pesticide poisoning in the municipality of Teresópolis - RJ. Rev. Econ Sociol Rural 2005; 43 (4)

Tomazin CC, Evaluation of first aid information on leaflets and pesticide labels according to sharecroppers in tomato plantations in Sumaré S.P Campinas: 2007 (Master's thesis - State University of Campinas)

Tordoir, WF & SITTERT, NJ. Organochlorines. Toxicology, 91: 51-57, 1994.

Trapé, AZ. Diseases Related to Pesticides: A Public Health Problem. Campinas: 1995 (Doctoral Thesis - State University of Campinas).

Trapé, A.Z. Toxicological Effects and Records of Pesticide Poisoning. Feagri/Unicamp , 2003. Available at : http://www.feagri.unicamp.br/tomates/pdfs/eftoxic.pdf. Accessed on:05/10/2008

Zambrone, FAD. Contribution to the study of poisoning in the Campinas region. Campinas: 1992 (Thesis - Doctorate - State University of Campinas).

CHAPTER 10

WORKS CONSULTED

Alavanja MCR, Hoppin Já, Kamel F 2004. Health effects of chronic pesticide exposure: cancer and neurotoxity. Annu Rev Public Health 25:157-197.

Benatto A. Health information systems for pesticide and related poisoning in Brazil: current situation and perspectives [Dissertation]. Campinas (SP): State University of Campinas; 2002.

Brazil, 1996 to 2001. National Toxic-Pharmacological Information System. Registered cases of human intoxication and poisoning. Available at http://www.cict.fiocruz.br. Accessed on: 05/04/2008.

Colosso C, Tiramani M & Maroni M 2003. Neurobehavioural effects of pesticides: state of the art. Neurotoxicology 24:577-591.

Faria, N.M., et al., Cross-sectional study on the mental health of farmers in the Serra Gaucha (Brazil). Revista de Saúde Pública, 33(4), 391-400, 1990.

FERNANDES,G. General classification of plaguicides. In: Intoxication by plaguicides: physiopathology, clinic and treatment. Montevideo, 1970. p. 151-161

FERNANDES,G. General classification of plaguicides. In: Intoxication by plaguicides: physiopathology, clinic and treatment. Montevideo, 1970. p. 211-283

Klein, C.H; Bloch, KV Sectional studies. In: Medronho, R.A; Carvalho, D.M; Bloch, K.V; Luiz, R.B; Wernick, G.L (Ed). Epidemiology I. São Paulo: Atheneu, 2006. p125 -150.

Peres F, Moreira JC & Dubois GS 2003. Pesticides, health and the environment: an introduction to the subject, pp. 21-41. In Is it poison or is it medicine? Pesticides, health and the environment. Fiocruz, Rio de Janeiro.

Silva JM et al. 1999. Familiar agriculture: production process and health conditions, p. 40. Proceedings of the XV World Congress on Safety and Health at Work. São Paulo, Brazil

Silva JM et al. 2005. Agrotoxics and work: a dangerous combination for the health of rural workers. Ciência e Saúde Coletiva 10(4) Rio de Janeiro Oct./Dec. 2005.

CHAPTER 11

ANNEXES

ANNEX I - Pesticide exposure investigation form

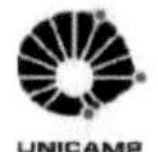

FACULTY OF MEDICAL SCIENCES DEPARTMENT OF PREVENTIVE MEDICINE ENVIRONMENTAL HEALTH PESTICIDE EXPOSURE INVESTIGATION FORM

1. Date: _____ ! ____ / _____

2. Name of Municipality: _______________________________________

3. Name of Health Unit: _______________________________________

CASE DATA

4. Patient's name: _______________________________________

5. Date of Birth: ___________ / ______ ! ____ **6. age:** (___________)

7. Sex: (______) 1-Male 2-Female 9-Unknown

8. Name of municipality of residence: _______________________________________

9. Zone: (___) 1.   Urban2-Rural

10. Neighbourhood: _______________________________________

11. Address, street, avenue, apartment no: _______________________________________

12. Reference Point: _______________________________________

13. Telephone (__) _______________________________________

14. Level of Education : (____)

    1-Unlearned 2-1st Grade 3-2nd Grade 4-Superior 5-Not applicable 9-Unknown

ADDITIONAL INFORMATION

15. Workplace: _______________________________________

16. Occupation: _______________________________________

17. Employment relationship: ( ) 1-Owner 2- Employee 3-Landlord/tenant

    4-Volante5-   Others6-   Not applicable

18. Job title :   (___)   1- Administrative 2- Agricultural Technician/Agronomist3-   Hose Puller

    4- Syrup Applicator/Preparer5-   Livestock Applicator

    6- Other7- _______________ Not applicable

19. Contact with pesticides:

How long have you been in contact with pesticides (poisons)? ________

Frequency of contact with pesticides: How many months a year? ________

________________ How many days a month? __________ or how many days a week? ____________ How many hours a day? ________________

When was the last time you had contact with __________ which product? _______________________

How do you apply the products?

( ) backpack pump   ( ) hose   ( )   tractor without cab

( ) tractor with closed cab   ( ) other (please specify): _______________________

20. Most commonly used pesticides

Trade Name	Active ingredient or toxicological class	34. Crops/ploughing

EPIDEMIOLOGICAL DATA

21. Main Exposure Route: (__________) 1-Cutaneous 2-Digestive 3-Breathing 4-Other: _______________

22. Have you had any poisoning? (Have you ever been sick from poison?) (__)   1- Yes 2- No

How often? (______)   1- Once only2-   More than once

Have you ever had to be hospitalised? (_)   1- Yes 2- No

How often? (______) 1- Once only2-   More than once

How long ago? (______) 1- Less than 10 years ago2-   More than 10 years ago

EPIDEMIOLOGICAL DATA ON CONTACT WITH PESTICIDES

23. Type of Contact : (_____) 1-Direct2-Indirect3-No Contact9-Neglected
Direct: direct handling, dilution and/or application; washing clothes used in application.
Indirect: planting, harvesting, weeding, packaging, pruning, trimming.

24. Personal Protective Equipment: 1-Yes 2-No 3-Not applicable 9-No **information**

(__)Long trousers (___)Long-sleeved shirt (___)Suitable waterproof clothing

(__)Closed toe shoes or boots ( )Suitable boots ( ) Gloves

(__)Goggles (________________)Mask (___)Hat (___)Cap (___) Ear protection

CLINICAL PICTURE

25. Smoking: 1-Yes2-No (___)Current (___)Previous

26. Alcoholism: 1-Yes2-No (___)Current (___)Previous

31. Pregnant woman: (_) 1-Yes 2-No3-Not Applicable9-Ignorant

32. Cardio Vascular Appt: 1-Yes 2-No9-Unknown

(_____) Hypotension (___________)Arrhythmia (___)Hypertension

33. Peripheral Central Nervous System: 1-Yes 2-No9-Ignorant

(___)Headache (___)Agitation/Irritability (___)Tremors

(___)Tingling in lower limbs (___)Tingling in upper limbs (___)Vertigo/dizziness

(___)Blurred vision (___)Decreased muscle strength (___)Motor incoordination

(___)Fasciculations

34. Digestive System : 1-Yes2-No9-Unknown

(___)Cramps (___)Diarrhoea (___)Nausea (___)Vomiting

(___)Epigastralgia (___) Heartburn ( )Burning

35. Respiratory System: 1-Yes 2-No3- Unknown

(___)Dyspnoea (_____) _________ Cough _______________ ( ) Bronchial secretion ( )Nasal irritation

36. Hearing aid: 1- Yes 2- No3- Ignored

( ) Hypoacusis ( ) Tinnitus

37. Skin and Mucosa: 1-Yes 2-No 9-Unknown

(___)Eye Irritation ________ ()Irritating DC (____)Sensitising DC

38. Urinary tract : 1-Yes 2-No 9-No information

(___)Decreased Flow / Oliguria (___)Dark Urine / Haematuria

LABORATORY DATA

39. CHOLINESTERASE TEST RESULT (EDSON METHOD) ________________ %

40. Referred to toxicology clinic: ( ) 1-Yes 2-No

Responsible for Customer Service ____________________________

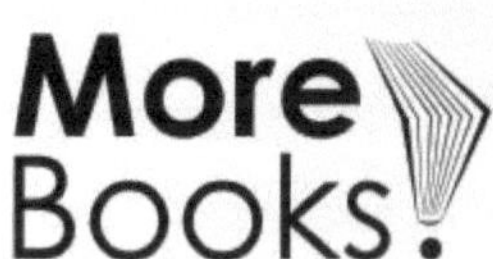

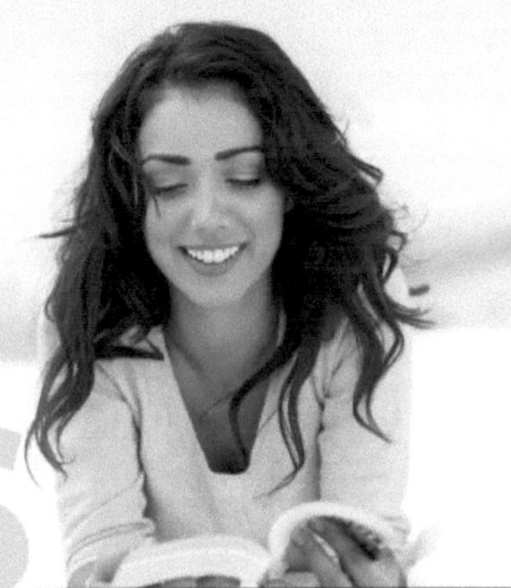

yes
I want morebooks!

Buy your books fast and straightforward online - at one of world's fastest growing online book stores! Environmentally sound due to Print-on-Demand technologies.

Buy your books online at
www.morebooks.shop

Kaufen Sie Ihre Bücher schnell und unkompliziert online – auf einer der am schnellsten wachsenden Buchhandelsplattformen weltweit! Dank Print-On-Demand umwelt- und ressourcenschonend produziert.

Bücher schneller online kaufen
www.morebooks.shop

info@omniscriptum.com
www.omniscriptum.com

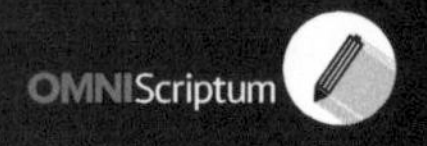

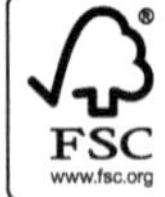

Printed by Books on Demand GmbH, Norderstedt / Germany